"When we pray,
GOD hears more
than we say,
HE answers more
than we ask,
HE gives more
than we imagine,
but....
In his own time,
In his own way!
So keep faith!!"

preet

A true story of faith, healing and love, God does hear us, he answers prayers, and he does heal. You must believe in order to have your prayers answered.

Ray Adkins

This book is dedicated to the following, for without them I would not be here writing this book.

Dr. Syed K Hasni, MD

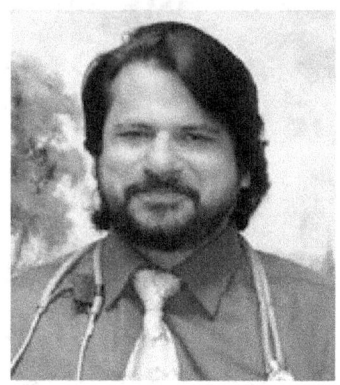

**My Doctor and friend.**

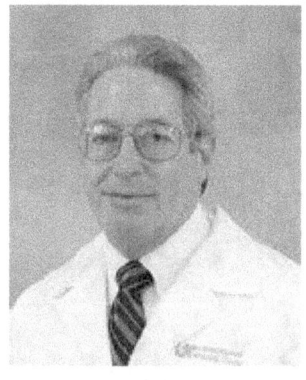

U.T Hospital
Frederick A. Klein, MD

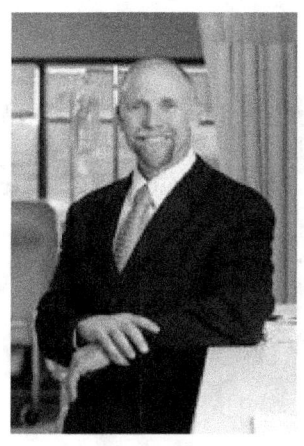

Mitchell Carl, M.D.
Hematology & Medical Oncology
Infectious Diseases Specialist

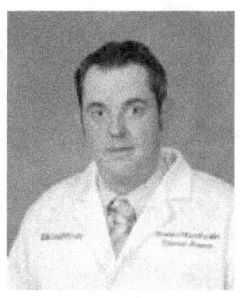

## U.K. Medical Center

Shane D. O'Keeffe, MD

**Vascular Surgeon**

And a very special thanks to:

My Lord Jesus Christ

My loving wife Debra J. Adkins

The staff and nurses at U.T. Hospital. Knoxville, Tenn.

The staff and nurses at St. Joseph Hospital, London, Kentucky.

The staff and nurses at U.K. Medical Center, Lexington, Kentucky.

The staff and nurses at Dr. Lohe and Hasni Office

The staff and nurses at Dr. Mitchell Carl's Office.

Cheryl Gibson, Physical Therapist

Angela Landrum, R.N.

My family and many friends, for without their prayers, love and affection, I never would have made it.

A true story of love, hope and faith, when faced with a crisis in health or any situation your faith in God will carry you through.

In my darkest time I called upon the Lord and he heard me, he still answers prayers and is in the healing business.

I am a living miracle of God, he picked me up and healed me in the pages to follow I will tell you how my dark time became light.

**"Know therefore that the LORD thy God, he is God, the faithful God, which keepeth covenant and mercy with them that love him and keep his commandments to a thousand generations."**

In order to be healed you must ask God to forgive you of your sins, and have mercy on you.

Prayer is the answer to all of our problems but we must believe in God and Love him with all our might. On the next page my story begins.

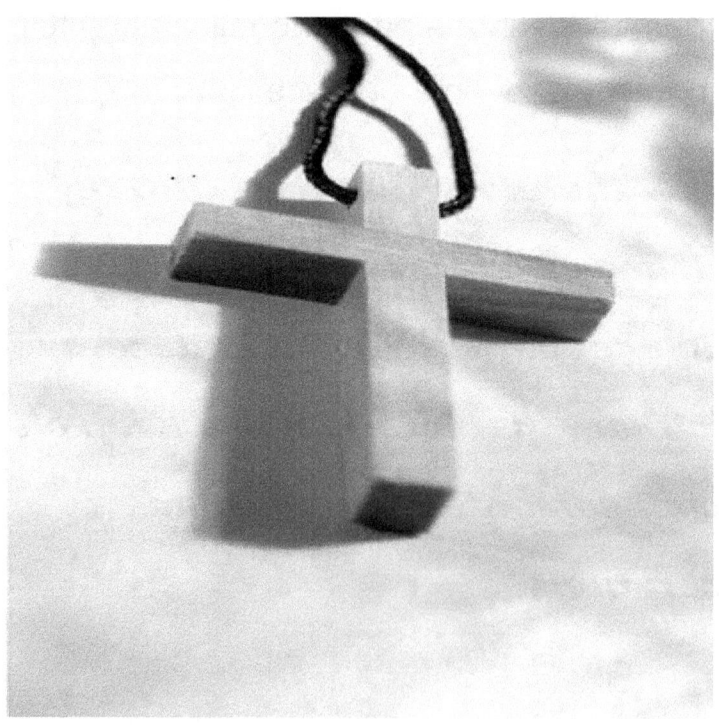

I am an average guy, married with two step children. I have worked all my life to survive and provide for my family. I am one of those people born without a silver spoon in my mouth. I have had to struggle, sacrifice, and scrape sometimes just to get by in life. I am not a rich man, but never considered myself poor either. I am just your average working guy who wants to enjoy a little bit of life if I can afford it. I served my country in the Military both in the Army and Navy. I served one year in Vietnam in 1972, and only come home with emotional scars, I considered myself lucky just to come home alive.

I never complained much about life in general; I just accepted the fact that is life and just make the best of it.

I have had some very good times and a few very bad times. I always managed to get by. I have worked for 36 years now and was looking forward to retiring and enjoying life. I knew that my ship sank somewhere or was hijacked because it never came in. I would have to live on what social security would pay, and I was willing to make the best of it. But, that was ten years away.

Life was going pretty decent now, and I enjoyed spending time with my wife and kids, even though they are grown now. I was content that everything was normal and we were paying our bills. I am 56 now and life is supposed to be better in this time in your life.

I work for the Knox County Board of Education for around three years now, as a custodian in the evening at Central Elementary.

I enjoy it very much, especially watching the children and have made some very good friends with the faculty, staff and the children too.

Then in May of 2010 things happened to me and my world changed forever.

**The LORD is my shepherd; I shall not want.**

**²He maketh me to lie down in green pastures: he leadeth me beside the still waters.**

**³He restoreth my soul: he leadeth me in the paths of righteousness for his name's sake.**

**⁴Yea, though I walk through the valley of the shadow of death, I will fear no evil: for thou art with me; thy rod and thy staff they comfort me.**

**⁵Thou 9repares a table before me in the presence of mine enemies: thou**

*anointest my head with oil; my cup runneth over.*

*[6]Surely goodness and mercy shall follow me all the days of my life: and I will dwell in the house of the LORD forever.*

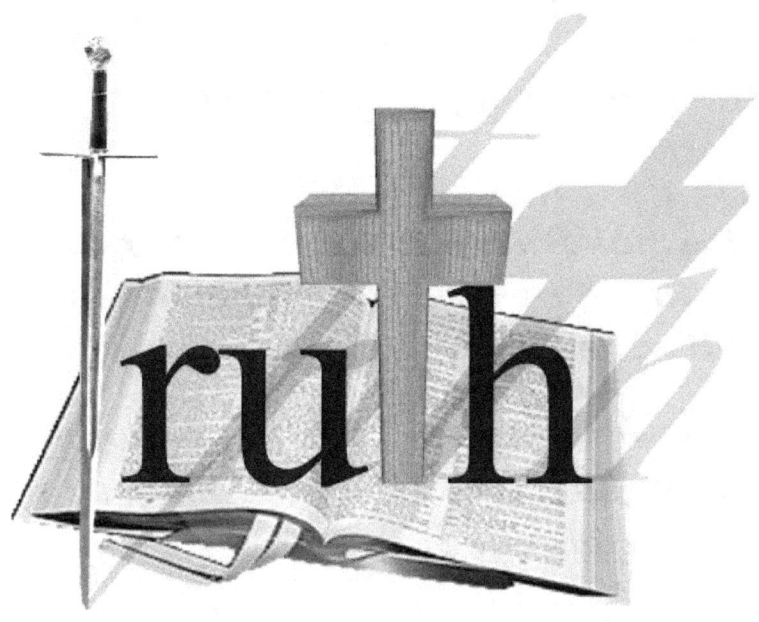

# Chapter One

## The Diagnosis

On or around the middle of May, I awoke one morning around 3:00 a.m. to urinate; I passed a lot of bright red blood and several big blood clots. I had made a mess in the bathroom and when my wife awoke around 7:00a.m. She had seen the blood. When I awoke I told her I needed to see the Doctor today. We got up and got ready and I went with her on the way to work (she works for my Doctor).

I told my doctor what had happened and sent me to the hospital for some lab work, and a C.T. scan. I had to wait a couple of days to get the results back.

Then one day my wife had gotten a copy of the report and brought it home for me to read. I knew she was upset at the way she was acting, I asked her was wrong and she said I had cancer in my bladder with a tumor inside and attached to my bladder wall. This was serious and my Doctor referred me to a Cancer Doctor in Corbin, Ky., a few miles away.

In the meantime my wife had made an appointment at the U.T. hospital to see a very good Urologist. I had an appointment on the same day to see the cancer Doctor then the Urologist the same day in the afternoon.

I have always been a religious man and attended church regularly, and prayed often. I prayed for some good news but, after speaking with the Cancer doctor I was told my cancer was in stage four, and the tumor had penetrated the bladder wall, and had wrapped itself around my artery in the pelvis region, and was growing quickly. The only recourse was probably radiation and my sentence on life was about three weeks of life left.

My heart sank and I told the doctor we were on our way to Knoxville, Tenn. to see the urologist. He stated it would be a waste of time, for no surgeon or anyone else could help me. On the way I thanked him for the diagnosis but I said" It is really not left up to you ". We headed out on our way to U.T. Hospital and I was making my will out, and I was concerned about my wife and my family.

I knew she was really worried, about my condition, and so was I. My heart was sad and I immediately went into prayer midway to Knoxville, I prayed very hard and all of a sudden I felt a touch like never before, a sensation not of this earth. I felt as if God himself had laid his hand on my shoulder and I tingled all over and relief came over me.

 I told my wife of the touch and our daughter Wendy who was driving, and my sister-in-law Zella, who went with us.

When we arrived at U.T.Hospital, I was in a much better state of relief than earlier. We made our way into the Doctors office and he did a cystoscope and said he thought he could remove the tumor, he said he may have to do two surgeries' to get it all out. He also said it did not appear to be cancerous. The appointment was made for two weeks later for the tumor removal.

I went home and did a lot of soul searching and on the date in two weeks seemed like it flew by.

I went in front of my church and asked for the anointing of oil.

This is what the Bible tells you to do.

**James 5:14-15) 14 Is any among you sick? Let him call for the elders of the assembly, and let them pray over him, anointing him with oil in the name of the Lord, 15 and the prayer of faith will heal him who is sick, and the Lord will raise him up. If he has committed sins, he will be forgiven**.

I was relived about doing this; I searched the scriptures for God's direction.

I am one of those people who does not ask for help, when I think I can do it myself. I just did not want to bother other people with my situation.

The next thing I knew it was time to go back to U.T. Hospital for the outpatient surgery.

# Chapter Two

## Outpatient Surgery

I arrived on June 3 rd to have my outpatient surgery. The Doctor was going to remove the tumor, and I would be able to go home that afternoon. The folks at U.T. Hospital were very compassionate and kind; I was treated very well from admission to pre-op surgery.

I joked without everyone trying to keep a positive attitude and made many of them smile. I have always had a sense of humor, and was not going to let this surgery get me down, besides God is with me.

I awoke and found myself in a hospital room with my wife and not in the outpatient room. I knew something had gone wrong.

Then the Doctor who had done my surgery came in and told me that he had gotten most of the massive tumor out of my bladder, but I had started bleeding and he had to stop. He suggested since it was so massive that I should consider having my bladder removed.

I told the Doctor he knew more than I and I would follow his advice, if that is what it took to get this behind me and get back to my life then so be it.

He made an appointment for me to return for a preview of what this would involve. I say many prayers a day but, I was focused on my situation and asked God to let his will be done. I am ready if it is my time to go; I am a winner either way where I go or if I stay. My main concern is my wife and family, I love them so much, and I knew if something happened to me they would be devastated.

My wife and I have been together for thirty years and I love her very much. I was concerned for her and not myself. What would she do if something happened to me?

My whole worldly life is centered around her; she is so precious to me. She is my best friend, lover, and companion and has made me the man I am today. She has helped me more than any one person in this entire world on many issues, and is someone I can talk to and trust with my life. We talk about everything, and we love each other and respect each other, she is a kind gentle, Christian woman. I tell her a hundred times during the day I love her.

**MARK 9:23**
**"'if you can'?" said Jesus. "Everything is possible for him who believes.**

I was at home and trying to prepare for idea of having my bladder removed. I was going to have to use a bag attached to my side to collect the urine in. I was told no one could tell I had the bag on under my clothes, where it would be located and all the instructions and etc that went with this procedure, and that I would be in the hospital for about five to nine days.

I was ready to get this to be behind me and hopefully this would be it, and my problems would be over .After a good cry at home while I was alone, I was determined to go ahead and do it. I am for whatever it takes, to do something if I don't like it, but if it is for the best then so be it.

**"In nothing be anxious, but in everything, by prayer and petition with thanksgiving, let your requests be made known to God."**

So when I did go back for my bladder removal I prayed that this would be it, even if I did have to wear a bag on my side, at least this would end the problem. The tumor would be gone and hopefully the cancer with it.

They prepared me for the major surgery and all was on schedule. I was satisfied in my decision and was going to stick to it. After all, I had Jesus and my wife with me. I was so proud of my wife who had been beside me the whole way, bless her heart she is tough.

When I awoke from this surgery again the doctor came in and informed me he could not remove the bladder because the tumor had wrapped around it and was choking my artery in my pelvis region. He said the only solution was chemotherapy and then come and see him when the chemotherapy was complete.

He stated he had removed several lympnodes for biopsy and I should have the results in several days. I was disappointed because none of the above surgeries had done me any good whatsoever. I accepted the fact that chemotherapy was imminent.

# Chapter Three

Chemotherapy here I come.

This I was afraid of, the word chemotherapy, I knew nothing about it, how it worked, how I was supposed to take it and etc. But, my wife while I was U.T. Hospital had them put in my upper left chest a thing called a porta-cath. This was supposed to make taking the I.V. type chemotherapy easier on me. With this device when they inserted the I.V. needles it would save my veins from being stuck so often.

My first visit for my chemotherapy I was scared to death, I did not understand it or anything. I have a very good Cancer Doctor in Corbin, Ky. I will refer to him as Dr. "C". When I arrived they showed me a movie on what chemo is, what it does and etc., which eased a lot of fears. Dr. "C" said I had to have six rounds of chemo.

I would take chemo for three days get a shot, and then return in two weeks. I just knew it was going to make me sick at my stomach, but, it did not. The only problem I have with chemo is the first day it takes seven hours to get my dose. The next two days about four to five hours, and the next day I get my shot, which builds my white cell count back up.

The nurses that work at Dr. "C"'s office are really not nurses they are angels, they are sweet ,kind, outgoing and very compassionate. For me, this is a true blessing, it is hard enough to have to take chemo, but, while under their care it eases the worry. I am on a first name basis with the nurses and I kind of look forward to going.

The chemo so far has not bothered me whatsoever; it is just a long visit and the office.

As of now I am in my fourth chemo treatment, and it is working. When I first started my cancer rating was 18.7 and now it is 2.5.

I was told that they rate cancer on a scale of 1-20. So see what God has done, my cancer is almost gone, Praise the Lord.

"For God does care for you, and loves you"

The only thing that has bothered me was the shot after the chemo, after the first shot it would cause my left foot to hurt, but the pain would come and go, and it was not that bad for it only lasted a short while. On my second round of chemo the shot caused my foot to hurt again and it lasted longer. After my third round my foot hurt and it went numb. I knew this was not good. I could not even walk, I had to hobble around, and it was not getting any better.

## Chapter Four

### To the hospital I go!

After my last shot, the numbness in my foot did not go away. My toes turned blue, and then back to the right color. I was worried then, but all this took place on the weekend, and the numbness would come and go. On Monday it was numb and stayed that way. My beloved Doctor Hasni called St. Joseph in London, Ky., and I was admitted to CCU.

My left foot hurt so bad I was in deep, severe pain, it felt as if someone was hitting my foot with a sledge hammer. The doctors came and went and they determined I had a blood clot just below my knee, which was blocking the circulation to my foot. They felt for a pulse in foot and there was none.

They put in a stent to try to get the circulation going again, but it failed. My foot was getting worse. During this stay my chemo was put on hold, I should have finished it on Nov 11, 2010.

They decided then maybe amputation just above the knee was the only way to solve the problem. By this time I was willing to do something, anything to get rid of the horrible pain I was experiencing. Dr, Hasni was not going to let that happen, he was determined to find another way to save my leg. He contacted a Doctor at U.K. medical center in Lexington, Kentucky.

I didn't want to go to U.K., I wanted to stay at St. Joseph, in London, Kentucky to stop the pain and do the amputation if necessary.

My wife insisted that going to U.K. was better and the doctors there just might save my leg. I decided to go, and after six days in London, I was U.K. bound. I was transported to U.K. via ambulance and admitted to U.K.

I met a Doctor O'Keeffe, and he told me that just maybe he could help my situation. I was transferred to ICU for a series of surgeries.

I under went four surgeries using a blood clot bursting medicine. I was admitted on Sunday and by Thursday I underwent the last of the procedures. I was tired of being in the hospital and all I could think of was home. I had many family and friends visit me in London and Lexington. I was so homesick; that it was all I could think of.

After the rounds of surgeries I was finally relived to have them over with, and my foot felt funny but it did not hurt, and I still had my leg and foot. I knew that God was watching over me and I knew he was there with me all along.

The time in the hospital was 15 days, it felt like 15 months, I drew closer to God during this time  and I enjoyed being closer to him, It was like I was on a first name basis's. I know that many prayers were offered to heaven by many churches, family and friends.

I have seen the works of the Lord in my life during these past several months; I knew he was healing me. I have seen with my own eyes the healing power of God, and felt his presence with me. It was truly a powerful feeling.

I prayed many a prayer during this ordeal concerning myself, my loving wife and family. I knew somehow my life was going to be different than ever before. I know now what is important and what is not. My days are more precious, my love for my God, my wife, my family and friends, is also more precious than ever before.

I am different in many ways now; I am more humble, thankful of the gift of healing. I truly love my Lord more than ever before. My love for him and my wife, family and friends, has more meaning.

I am walking now on my leg they wanted to amputate, my foot is healing, and my chemo continues. I want to especially thank my wife, who stood by me the whole time during my ordeal; she was beside me the whole way.

I cannot thank her enough for the love and kindness she has shown me. I have the best wife in the whole wide world.  I am so thankful to God for sending her to me. I love her so much, and with my whole heart.

My last pet scan came back as stable after missing two months of Chemo. I am continuing with the last two sessions which should end the first week of January 2011.

The Lord has truly blessed me, a big special thanks to Barbara, Tracy, Lisa, Callie, Kelly, Liz and Karen, I love you all very much, thanks for your love and compassion.

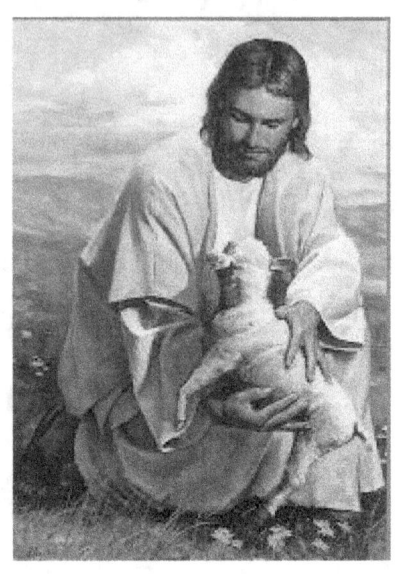

He will never forsake us.

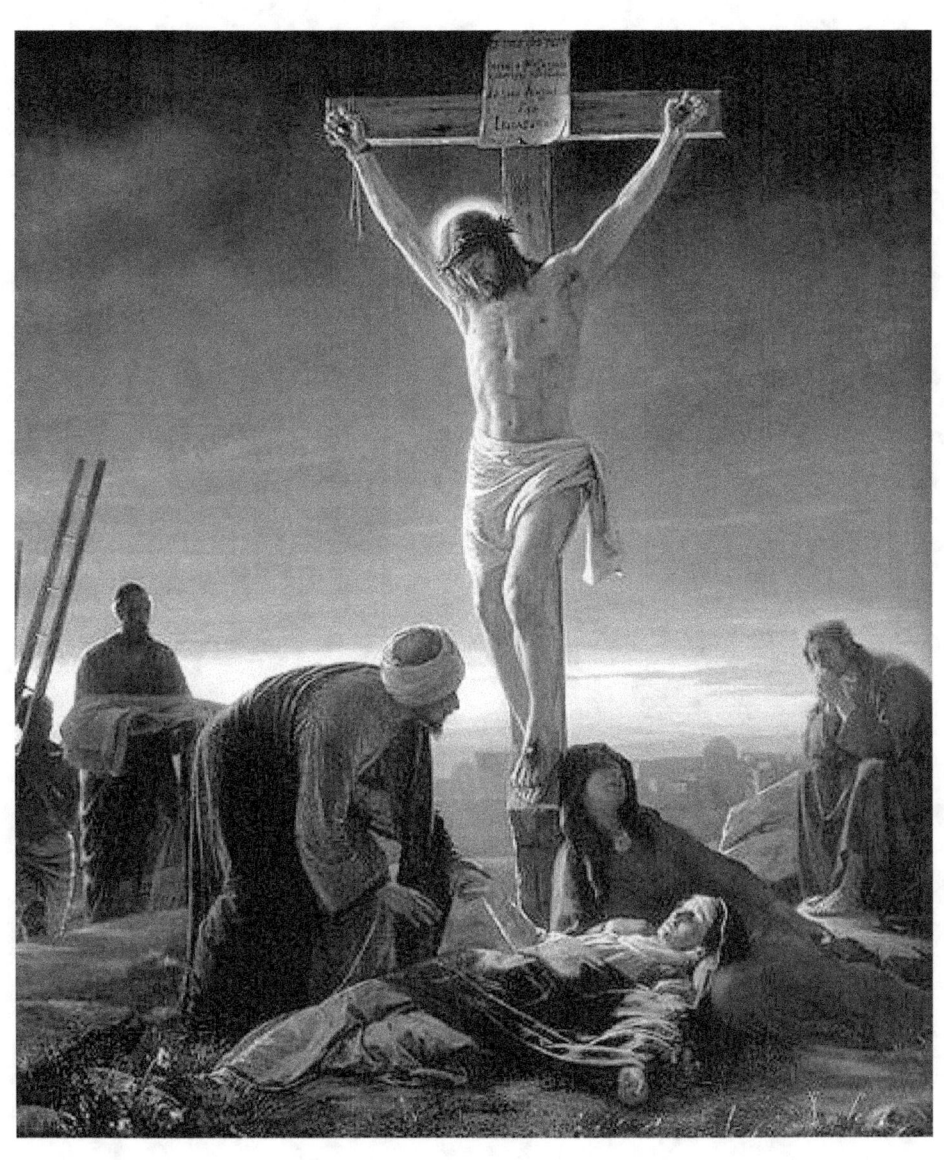

www.ingramcontent.com/pod-product-compliance
Lightning Source LLC
Chambersburg PA
CBHW071320280526
45788CB00004B/1964